Arthritis Explained

Arthritis Overview, Causes, Types, Management, Prevention, Treatments, Effects, Symptoms, Causes and Much More!

By Frederick Earlstein

Copyrights and Trademarks

Disclaimer and Legal Notice

Foreword

A debilitating disease, arthritis has been serving up all sorts of pain in women, children and men; arthritis affects millions of people all over the world. A condition in which one or more joints of a person swells up causing stiffness and joint pains. This condition is a painful disease that can be caused by underlying medical conditions or from a sustained injury. Arthritis typically becomes worse with the onset of maturity and has become the bane of many people living with the disease. There are at least a hundred forms and sorts of arthritis and with so many of them; it is sometimes difficult to zero in on the cause in order to find out a solution to manage the pain.

Arthritis typically entails and brings about stiffness and joint pain that can exceed the limits of pain a person can endure. It can go beyond the actual physical symptoms and can be caused by a myriad of things. Because arthritis can originate from over a hundred forms of joint diseases, it is the leading cause of disability in the United States and the greater North American countries. Although arthritis has been identified as the culprit of many pains and aches that plagues, women, children and men of varied ages, there is still much left about the disease that needs to be understood and discovered.

The disease can suddenly become apparent and mimic other diseases, thereby defying treatment. The symptoms of the disease is clear, the pains felt by those suffering from it can't deny it - however, more frequently than not the discomfort and pain that comes along with arthritis will not manifest itself on the surface of the body. Hence, we have compiled an informative little booklet that would help you determine the reasons and causes for the disease that immobilizes many today. From the most common form of arthritis that has been diagnosed to the more complex origins of the disease, the jury is in - there is undoubtedly a slew of sources that could be the reason for why people are subject to the debilitating disease.

We shall be talking about the most common, and not so common, forms of arthritis in this book and attempt to shed more light in the otherwise difficult to determine roots of the disease.

All the different forms of arthritis can be the cause and reason of why the lives of many people are compromised in terms of mobility. The quality of life of a person suffering from the disease can range from tolerable aches to excruciating, life-changing pain. Joint swelling and inflammation is how arthritis manifests itself, and with more than over a hundred types of arthritis that has been identified, it can be a daunting task to determine the actual cause in order to receive that proper treatment and administer the proper form of pain management.

Different forms of arthritis seem to attack one person or another, depending on their risk factors. It is a choosy disease that homes in on individuals for their physiology and make, with women being more susceptible to one form of the disease and men being targeted by another. It is an opportunistic disease can cause widespread symptoms and affect multiple organs, and affects a large part of the world population including children.

Table of Contents

Chapter One: Arthritis in Focus

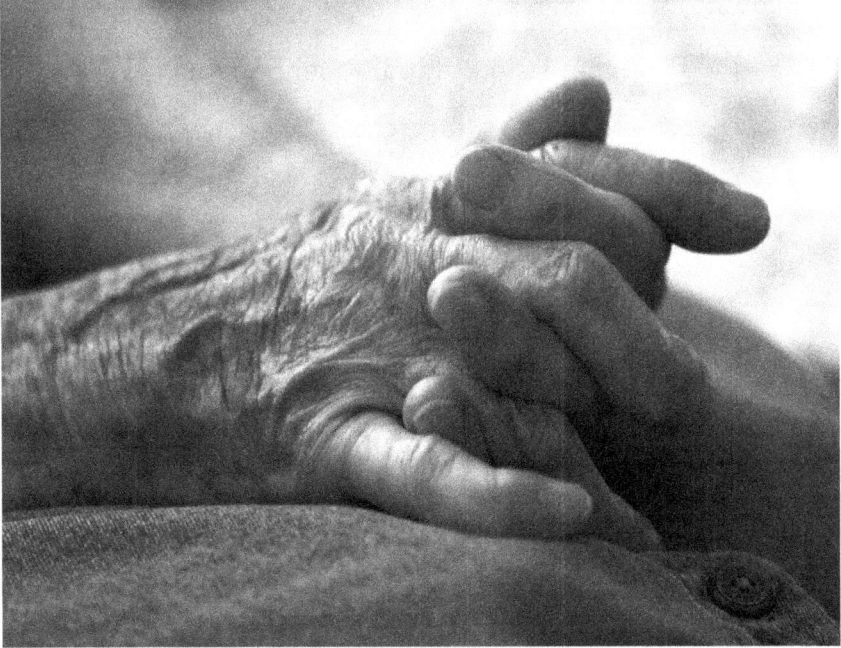

Medical science and experts of the disease have identified about two hundred forms of rheumatic conditions and diseases which affect the joints of an individual suffering from arthritis. The alarming bit about arthritis is that it can affect not only the joints of a patient; it can also involve the various internal organs of an individual and impair the immune system of the body. The Center for Disease Control and Prevention in the United states have determined a staggering 54.4 million adults who have been diagnosed with the debilitating condition that is reason for the immobilization of a big chunk of the population the country. Although arthritis is believed to be more apparent and widespread in individuals over 65 years old, children and young people are not spared of the disease. It can affect anyone, young or old.

The symptoms of arthritis not only has the patient experiencing pain it can also literally stop one in their tracks and immobilize them because of the pain that comes along with the disease, resulting in the deterioration of their quality of life. Many people who suffer through the physical pain of the symptoms of arthritis also go through mental turmoil, because of the effects of the pain that not only limits but inhibits their daily activities and preventing them from earning a living, contributing positively to society, or exploring new avenues they would have otherwise been able to enjoy.

The factors that contribute to the development of arthritis can stem from the abnormal metabolism of an individual; therefore proper diagnosis is crucial to discovering the origins of the disease in order for treatment to zero in on the intended target. It can also come from a host of infections and from the dysfunction of a person's immune system. Arthritis can also detected back to the genetic makeup of a person making an individual whose family has history of the disease, more prone to the condition that lowers the quality of life of the individual.

A patient suffering from swollen joints and joint pains will need to get the expertise of a specialist in order to determine the origins of the symptoms so as to get the proper treatment that would target the cause and reason of the disease. Treatment aims to control the pain a patient suffers and there are, thankfully, a number of avenues a patient can take in terms of pain management. With proper diagnosis and the right treatment administered, the chances of a patient suffering from arthritis can greatly improve their quality of life and curb further deterioration. The possible treatments available to a patient (depending on the diagnosis of the arthritis) range from the administering of medications to non-pharmacological therapies.

Treatment of a patient with arthritis can include physical or occupational therapy, which encourages rehabilitation of the patient through the carrying out of specific activities needed in their daily life.

In some cases, patients are recommended to go on supervised, specific exercise regimens that would serve as an initial step to recovery and wellness. But in some cases, arthritis patients who exhibit more severe forms of the disease may be advised to use assistive tools and aids that allow them for better mobility. Splints, canes, walkers, and braces, are just some of the tools some patients are advised to use alongside pharmacological medication. Surgery is the ultimate recommendation for arthritis patients whose disease is far too serious and grave for medication and therapy to combat. Let's delve a little deeper and get to know more about what can be done to arrest arthritis before it gets any worse.

Risk Factors of Arthritis

It is difficult to pinpoint the factors that cause arthritis just by looking at an affected area alone. Most times, especially during the onset of the disease, there are no telltale signs that would give indication of the disease. There is no single culprit of all the sorts of arthritis determined by medical science, but there are in fact a host of reasons and causes for the ailments development. Depending on the sort or form of arthritis, the causes of the illness being present in an individual are varied. Just as the causes are varied, so are the symptoms since some can be more severe than other forms.

A person undergoing the development of arthritis could be suffering from the disease because of **abnormal metabolism**. When a person's metabolism is out of whack, the anomaly can lead to gout or pseudogout. Another cause of arthritis can stem from an injury sustained which could develop into more severe complications like **degenerative arthritis**. Osteoarthritis is a condition that can be passed on through the genes of an individual - when a family has a history of osteoarthritis, the chances of an individual from that family developing arthritis exponentially heightens.

Lyme disease, a disease born of a tick bite is also a cause for painful arthritis in a patient. The varied list of reasons and causes of arthritis can run at an arm's length and beyond, therefore in order to receive the proper treatment to arrest, or at the very least, manage the pain, a proper investigation of the history of the patient will be vital.

Chapter Two: The Symptoms of Arthritis

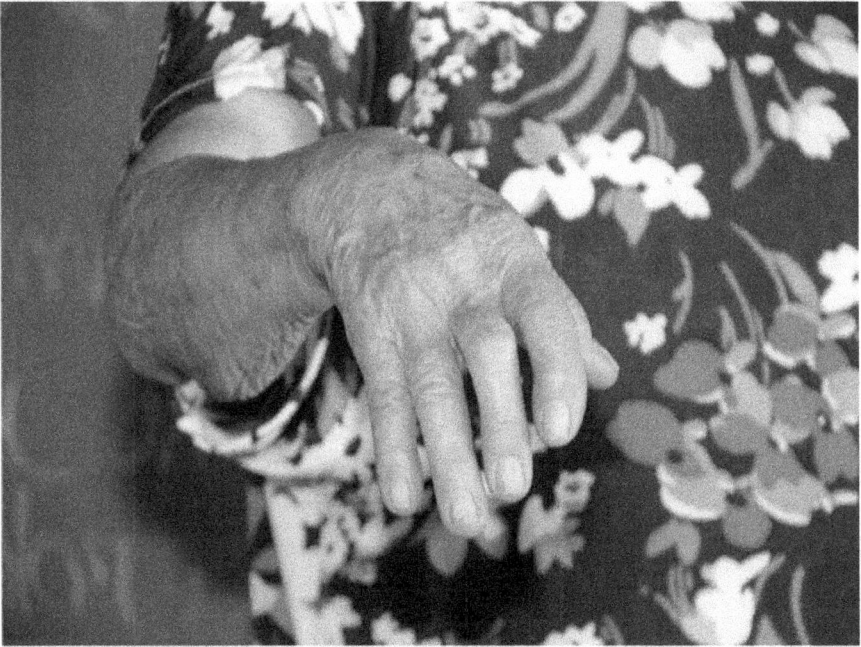

Inflammations of the joints occur in patients at the onset and the development of arthritis. Inflammation is a process the body goes under wherein the body's white blood cells along with its immune protein assist in giving us protection from foreign elements such as viruses and bacteria. This is how our bodies help in shielding us from infections. However, in some diseases, the immune system of a person, or its defense system, sets off an inflammatory signal even when forcign substances are absent.

Conditions as these are called autoimmune diseases. This is when the immune system creates havoc over its own tissues responding as if healthy tissues were in a state of infection. Misdirected inflammation is the outcome of some types of arthritis like Psoriatic arthritis, rheumatoid arthritis, gout, and systemic lupus erythematosus. Let's take a look at the symptoms of these two most commonly diagnosed types of arthritis.

Common Symptoms

Also known as rheumatoid disease is one sort of inflammatory arthritis that is accompanied by chronic joint swelling. It typically manifests on the joints of an arthritic patients hands, knees, feet, and hands. Rheumatoid arthritis affects the entire system impacting the body's organs. Patients who suffer from rheumatoid arthritis experiences a myriad of physical symptoms such as swelling, redness, tenderness, warmth and stiffness of the patient's joints causing severe pain. The motion and movability of the joints are compromised making the patient compensate on their movements by limping. More than one joint is usually involved. If left unchecked and untreated joints will begin to show deformity and the proper function and task of the joint/s diminishes. Rheumatoid arthritis is also accompanied by fatigue, fever, and anemia.

Fatigue

Fatigue is a common symptom of rheumatoid arthritis and is most especially felt by the suffering patient when there is active inflammation of the joints. The body responds to the effects of the disease resulting in poor sleep quality brought about by pain. Fatigue is the body's way of reacting to the inflammation experienced by the patient's joints. It can also be brought about by the body's reaction to medication. Because of the limited mobility and calculated movements of the patient, the fatigue an individual suffering from RA can be overwhelming. This spirals to changes and sudden shifts in moods, relationships suffer, occupation and productivity is disrupted because the attention of the suffering patient is averted from the necessary task.

Creativity can come to a standstill and the happiness quotient of the suffering patient is at a low. It is not unusual for those suffering from the ailment to display weight loss due to poor appetite.

Joint Pains

Joints pains are apparent with people suffering from RA. The joints of the suffering patient swell up when the disease is active and in full swing. It is not unusual for inflammation to also take place should the joints already have suffered previous damage. When rheumatoid arthritis is active, it paves the way for the joints to swell up because of the lining tissue of the joint thickening and also to the excess joint fluid present in the localized area. When this transpires, the swollen joint expands and stretches out, irritating the capsule that encloses the joint. The capsules of our joints are fitted with nerve endings that send pain signals to the brain.

A patient previously diagnosed with RA can experience and suffer permanent deterioration of the joint, damaging the cartilage, ligaments and bones of the suffering individual - this will then cause extreme pain and utter discomfort when the joint needs to be utilized.

Tenderness and Loss of Range of Motion

It is not uncommon for RA to lead to tenderness experienced in the joints of the suffering patient. The affected and inflamed joint lining tissue attacks and irritates the nerves in the joint capsule resulting in pain and tenderness. When this happens, the joint capsule is compressed by external pressure, and is felt through touch or when weight/pressure is placed on the area. The pain felt is immediate and excruciating. Movement is not only limited because of the pain it is constrained as well because of the amount of pain and discomfort. This is why people suffering from RA often, at the very least suffer from interrupted sleep and at its extreme, insomnia.

The joints affected by RA become increasingly inflamed if not treated, and this leads up to the incomplete range of motion for the region affected. When loss of joint range of motion is present, weakness of the areas involved is reported. When left unchecked, undiagnosed and untreated, deterioration is inevitable and loss of range of mobility can become permanent.

Swelling and Stiffness

Patients with RA have one thing in common and that would be the presence of swollen joints. The swelling of the joints can range from mild to extreme. People who suffer from RA can usually tell when their joints are swollen because it is not only apparent through sight; it is also felt by the individual. When the joints of the RA sufferer are in full swing, it makes it harder for the individual to move due to the loss of range of mobility on the affected area. Stiffness of the joints or difficulty in mobility and movement is another symptom of RA. This is when the joints affected by active RA are swollen and stiff.

Stiffness of the joint is usually more apparent and felt in the morning rather than any other time of the day. Physicians will inquire about the length of time the stiffness is felt by the patient, allowing them insight that gives clue to the gravity of the active joint inflammation. The duration of morning stiffness of the joints diminishes as the RA responds to treatment given.

Redness and Warmth

Aside from the apparent swelling of the joints when the RA is active, redness also is seen in the localized regions affected. The capillaries of the skin over the inflamed region widens due to the nearby inflamed joints of the area. The widened capillaries, also called dilated capillaries exacerbate the situation and display it apparent. When the affected joints of the patient are inflamed and the RA is active, the joints are warm to the touch. Response to treatment usually addresses the joint warmth. There are cases and instances when there is no apparent redness or swelling, but warmth is felt in the localized region affected by RA.

Rheumatoid arthritis typically affects many small joints of the wrists and hands. It also typically affects the balls of the patient's feet. It is not uncommon to detect RA to affect other parts of the patient's body like their hips, shoulders, knees, and ankles. When this happens the affected areas become swollen, tender, warm and painful. The occurrence of more than four joints being affected is called polyarthritis. A few affected joints, when inflamed are called oligoarthritis and a singular inflamed joint is referred to as monoarthritis.

Deformity of Joints

Chronic rheumatoid arthritis can result to joint deformity in the suffering patient. When left unchecked and untreated, inflammation of the areas affected leads up to the deterioration of the cartilage and bone whilst loosening the ligament of the affected region. When left unchecked, permanent joint deformity and ruin will occur.

Limping

Compromised lower extremity function due to RA is made apparent by the patient's limited and labored mobility. Limping could be caused by a number of other ailments of the muscles, bones and nerves. However, in RA affected individuals, the malaise targets the hips, knees, ankle or feet of the individual. A noticeable limp exhibited by the individual is caused by extreme pain and discomfort, a loss of range of motion of the affected areas, and is accompanied by swelling of the joint. Young children are not exempt from the symptoms of RA.

Chapter Three: Common Forms of Arthritis

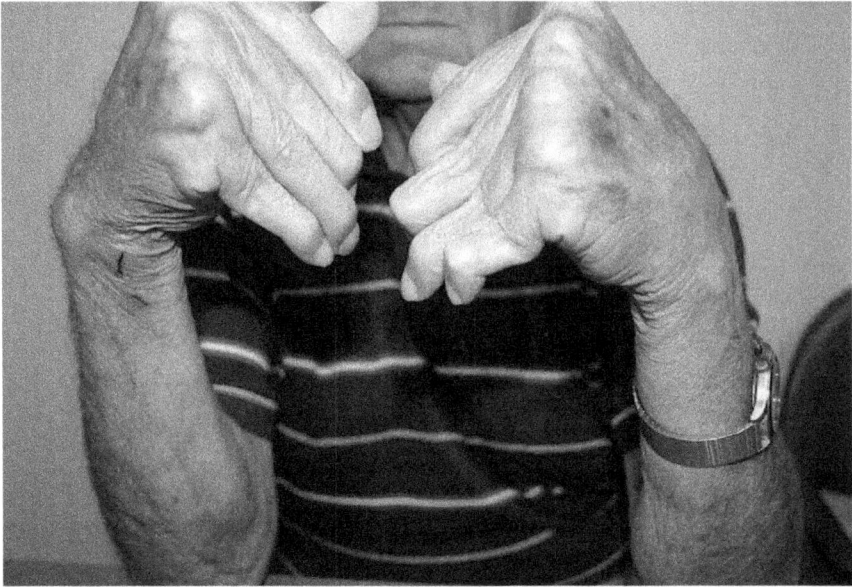

There are varied causes and different forms of arthritis and the symptoms and pain that comes along with the disease can be anywhere from mild to incapacitating. Observation and studies have resulted in findings that determine specific kinds of arthritis which men, women and children report. With over a hundred forms of arthritis and with the lifestyle of present days, it is no wonder that we see over 54 million people in suffer the painful disease. Our bodies are comprised of hundreds of bones that are joined by the clear, slick cover on each end ot the tip of the joint.

When the protective and lubricated film at the tips of the joints erode deteriorates, the nerve endings are exposed and the tips of the affected joints begin rubbing against each other.

Rheumatoid Arthritis

This form of arthritis is classified as an autoimmune disease wherein the immune system of the individual suffering from the disease attacks parts of the body, zeroing in on the joints of the individual. When the immune systems attacks the joints, the affected joints of the patient become swollen and this can eventually lead to damage of the joints if left untreated.

Rheumatoid nodules are bumps that develop on the skin of 1 out of 5 RA patients. These typically show up in the areas where the joints that handle pressure are located like the elbows, heels and knuckles of a person. Rheumatoid arthritis is a disease that still stumps doctors and specialists because they have not been able to figure out what causes the disease.

Experts are still divided on the causes of rheumatoid arthritis, with some supposing that the immune system becomes confused after a bout with infection, begins to attack the joints of the affected individual. This, when it happens, can spread to the rest of the body. On the other hand, researchers and scientists suppose that two chemicals in the body which are associated with inflammation - tumor necrosis factor (TNF) and interleukin-1, set off other components of the immune system. This being said, there are drugs that help block these chemicals from attacking the body, improving the symptoms of rheumatoid arthritis and preventing further joint damage.

The symptoms of rheumatoid arthritis are frequently more severe than that of osteoarthritis and the symptoms can suddenly show and feel apparent, or these symptoms can come slowly over time. Patients usually complain of stiffness and pain, reporting the sensation of their joints feeling "fused" together. The stiffness, swelling and pain is usually felt in the wrists and/or hands, the elbows and/or shoulders, the knees and/or ankles, the feet, jaw and/or neck of the patient.

Rheumatoid arthritis usually affects more than one joint and is apparent in multiple joints of the suffering individual. The symmetrical pattern of the attacks of rheumatoid arthritis is common, meaning that if one side of the body experiences swelling and pain, the counterpart on the other side of the body will also experience the same. Another indication of the disease, apart from the swelling and pain that come along with the condition, is the warm sensation felt in the area affected by rheumatoid arthritis.

Swelling of the joints does not dissipate and can get in the way of usual daily and mundane tasks such as driving, walking, working, sweeping, standing, stooping, squatting (if you work on a garden). Even opening twist cap bottles and jars can be challenging for a person suffering from rheumatoid arthritis.

The sensation of feeling stiff would usually be the most pronounced during the morning, upon waking up and could last for the good part of the day, making it difficult for the patient suffering from it go about their usual chores and job. These patients would complain of fatigue and display a continued spell of a lack of appetite resulting in the patient's weight loss. Rheumatoid arthritis is opportunistic and could affect not only the joints of the individual; it can also have serious effects on the heart, lungs and eyes of the patient

Osteoarthritis

The second most commonly reported form of arthritis suffered by people the world over is osteoarthritis and it affects millions. Osteoarthritis happens when the cartilage that protects and covers the ends of the bones erode and wear down over time. This condition can be present anywhere in the patient's body but is most commonly seen affecting the joints of the hands, knees, hips and spine. The symptoms of this ailment can typically be managed effectively through treatment, therapy and medication (or the combination of two or all methods of management) but the process, once it has begun, is usually irreversible. Methods to manage the condition, and to assist in slowing down the progression of the disease, include staying physically active, regulating and maintaining appropriate weight (hence lessening the impacts on the affected areas), allowing for better joint function and lessening the chances of immobilizing pain.

The causes of osteoarthritis is the gradual deterioration of the cartilage which cushions the ends of the bones of the joints - when this happens both ends of the bones essentially meet and rubs up against each other therefore causing pain when or after you move. It is accompanied by tenderness in the region affected when light pressure is applied. You will notice a stiffness of the joints upon getting up in the morning or after a spell of inactivity. People who suffer from this disease find it difficult to move and get out of bed, especially after waking up. A grating sound or sensation when the bone is used is another strong indication of the degenerative disease.

Often times, the damage caused by the grating of the bones pave the way for the body to develop bone spurs to "compensate" for the gap. These feel like hard lumps which may develop around the joints affected by osteoporosis.

When the cartilage, the firm and lubricated tissue which allows our joints frictionless motion and acts as a cushion that protects the ends of our bones in the joints slowly wears away, the affected joints rub grate against each other, signaling the brain and transmitting the message to pain receptors. The lubricated part of the surface of the cartilage then shows wear and becomes rough and infirm. When the wear down of the cartilage is complete the bone to bone rubbing makes for painful movement and limited mobility.

Research has shown that the risk of osteoarthritis heightens with the onset of age. As people mature and their bodies show wear and damage, the greater the risk. Though it is not clear why, it appears that more women than men are likelier to develop the disease.

The extra body weight of an individual can also be a reason of the wear down of cartilages. The more a person weighs, the higher the likelihood of the developing the disease since the extra weight gives additional stress to the joints which bears weight on the joints. The fat tissue then creates harmful proteins which cause the swelling in and around the joints of the area. When a person gets injured, whether from sports or an accident, the chances of osteoarthritis in that individual also increase. Past injuries that a patient may have healed from still and also make them a candidate for the disease.

Other considerations and risk factors that increase the chances of osteoarthritis in a person is their occupation. When a task requires a person to take repetitive stress on a particular and localized area of a joint, that joint may end up developing the disease. Even genetics is a factor in the risk of developing osteoarthritis. A person is more predisposed to developing the disease if it has been present in other family members. Osteoporosis has a way of finding its way down a family tree.

A person born with damaged cartilage or malformed joints are also more susceptible to osteoarthritis. When ignored and put off for later, this degenerative disease will worsen making it more difficult to manage; therefore it is important to get checked by a physician immediately. Severe pain can make even the most mundane of daily tasks, such as physically getting out of bed, difficult, painful and frustrating. Early detection and diagnosis gives the patient a better chance of managing the disease, lifestyle changes, medication, and therapy can help.

Symptoms of the disease usually develop gradually and worsen over time. Physical indications of osteoarthritis include pain in the joints while in motion or after movement. Tenderness of the joint affected is apparent when light pressure is applied to the area in question. Stiffness of the joint is most apparent upon waking in the morning; stiffness may also be apparent to the patient suffering from the disease after a period of inactivity. The loss of flexibility on the affected area is seen, and the full range of motion is depleted.

Another symptom of the disease is the grating sensation the patient reports when the joint is utilized. Bone spurs, or extra bone bits that form around the affected joints, feel like hard lumps. When these are felt and manifest in an individual it is strongly advised that the patient make an appointment to see the doctor.

Chapter Four: Other Types of Arthritis

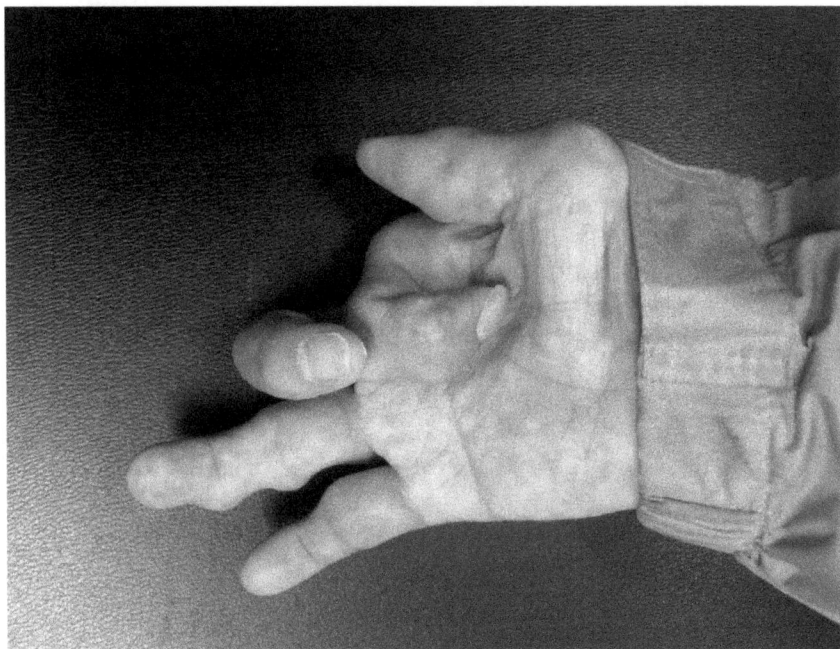

There are over a hundred kinds of arthritis that an individual can be prone to whether it is because of the lifestyle they lead or passed down from one generation to the next. With so many sorts of this disease, it can be difficult to tell which sort of arthritis a person is suffering from. In order to determine what kind of arthritis one has, there is quite a bit of asking and reading up to be done. Let's take a closer look at some of the more common ones that people of various ages and genders complain of in this section.

Psoriatic Arthritis

Psoriasis arthritis limits the range of motion of the patient affected. They experience stiffness and tenderness of the joint. They experience bouts of pain caused by the condition. It is not uncommon for patients with psoriatic arthritis to notice their nails changing, an example would be pitting, and this is noticed in about 8-% of psoriatic arthritis patients. Roughly a third of patients suffering from psoriasis will most likely also develop psoriatic arthritis.

The condition typically targets individuals between the ages of 30 to 50 years of age. However, it is not unusual to acquire the condition at any stage of life. This condition mainly affects the joints of the individual, causing the affected areas to become inflamed.

In order to determine if it is indeed psoriatic arthritis a person has, a doctor will have to order tests to prove its occurrence. Patients suffering from psoriatic arthritis would often notice swelling in their knees, feet, ankles, and hands.

It typically manifests itself through the joints causing them to swell. The joints would then get very painful and puffed up. The affected joints would feel hot to the touch and looks like angry red welts. The fingers and toes of a patient affected with psoriatic arthritis would puff up and look like swollen sausages. Joints are painfully stiff in the morning making it difficult for the patient to move. It has a tendency to attack joints in pairs, mirroring the condition of one side of the body and expressing it on the other. It is typical to experience psoriatic arthritis in both knees, both ankles, both elbows and either side of the hips. Stiffness and pain in the neck, the upper and lower back, as well as the buttocks may stem from the swelling in the joints of the spine and the hip bones of the patient, making movement and mobility painful and limited.

Psoriatic arthritis is a rare disease as it is utterly damaging. The destruction caused by this form of arthritis quickly damages the joints of the patient at the tips of their toes and fingers rendering them useless. When this happens, and the joints cease to operate in the manner they are meant to, the patient can run into all sorts of challenges like keeping their balance. It would pose difficult for a person with deteriorated joints in their toes to stand or walk and it likely that a person suffering from psoriatic arthritis to have trouble utilizing their hands the way they are meant to be used.

The tendons of the psoriatic arthritis patient could also become affected through time. The muscle that connects to a bone could become inflamed causing pain with moving such as when needing to climb or alight stairs. Tiny dents and ridges, called pitting, are apparent on the nails of both hands and feet of the patient with psoriatic arthritis. The eyes too can become affected, making the colored portion of the eye; this can be very painful when exposed to bright light. Although rare, shortness of breath accompanied by chest pains can be some of the symptoms a patient with psoriatic arthritis feels. This happens when the chest wall and the cartilage joining your ribs to the breastbone becomes inflamed making it difficult to take easy breaths.

On even rarer occasions, the lungs or the aorta, which are the large blood vessel that exits the heart can be affected by psoriatic arthritis. Anyone diagnosed with psoriasis who experience painful hands will have to get seen by a physician immediately because of the higher likelihood of the patient developing psoriatic arthritis Patients may also get psoriatic arthritis even though they have not been diagnosed with psoriasis therefore any individual experiencing painful and/or swollen joint, irritated eyes and stiffness in the joints should head to see the doctor as soon as possible.

Early detection and an accurate and timely diagnosis of the condition will alleviate further damage and any deformity that would eventually prevent proper movement and ease of mobility. Expect the physician to give you a physical examination asking about symptoms you are feeling. The doctor will also be inquiring about your family's medical history as well as your own. You will be given a series of lab test in order for the doctor to get a better insight of what is happening inside of you.

Imaging, scanning and blood exams will help the doctor make a proper diagnosis. Because psoriatic arthritis looks a lot like rheumatoid arthritis, it will be likely that your physician will want to give additional tests to rule this out. The most telling indications of the disease are the skin and nail transformations that accompany psoriasis. Telling changes in one's X-rays will also give indication. A condition that usually rears around to ages of 30 to 50, psoriatic arthritis can also affect a young person.

Psoriatic arthritis can also manifest itself through red, itchy blotches on the skin. It also manifest on the skin as thick, gray, scale like protrusions. And because it can also affect the eyes of a person, there may be some swelling and redness that is apparent to a patient. Psoriatic arthritis and psoriasis are gene-related conditions that can be passed down from one generation to the next, therefore it is best to see a doctor when an individual notices or feels any of the symptoms that come along with the condition.

Gout

Gout is a sort of arthritis which results in a sudden swelling of affected joints. This condition is developed by uric acid crystals being deposited in the affected joint and can cause symptoms such as the appearance of nodules beneath the skin (tophi). A patient suffering from gouty arthritis would notice warmth, redness and swelling of the joints accompanied by joint pains. One effective manner of diagnosing the condition is for fluid to be extracted from the affected region and examined by use of a microscope to see if there is uric acid crystals present in the extracted fluid.

When gouty arthritis is left unchecked and undiagnosed, there is no way for proper treatment to be administered. If not diagnosed early and given proper medication and treatment, gouty arthritis can lead to irreversible damage to the affected joints, tophi and kidney damage, acute attacks of gouty can stem from dehydration, surgery, beverages high with sugar content or high fructose corn syrup. It can be triggered as well by alcoholic beverages such as beer, and other liquor. Gouty arthritis can also be triggered by consuming large and frequent amounts of red meat and seafood.

Patients who are diagnosed with gouty arthritis are strongly advised to change their diet and limit all foods and beverages that trigger the flare ups and swelling episodes that accompany the condition. Patients diagnosed with gouty arthritis are recommended to stay away from consuming too much fish, shellfish and seafood including sardines scallops mackerel anchovy codfish mussel's herring haddock and trout. Other meats such as bacon video turkey venison beef kidney Liver and sweetbreads are also to be avoided.

The signs and symptoms of gout typically affect one joint. The pain that the patient feels is usually very severe and is reflective of the Seriousness of the swelling in the joint. The affected area is tender and warm to the touch and there are some instances when even the slightest movement or brushing of object against it causes excruciating pain.

Joint effusion is the term to describe excessive fluid deposited in the affected area of the body. Gout usually affects the joints of the lower extremities of the patient's body usually are getting the big toe. This is a condition of gout the atrocities that is called podagra. However it is also not unusual for other parts like the photo knee ankle and elbow wrist hands and other joints of the body to be affected by gout. When gout is long-standing and severe it can affect multiple joints all at once causing joint stiffness and excruciating pain in multiple joints of the patient's body.

Gout can also be recognized through the presence of tophi. This is a hard nodule of uric acid that is concentrated under the localized affected area of the skin. It can show a parent in different regions of the patient's body typically on the patients elbow's on the upper ear cartilage or on other surface joints. When tophi nodules are present, these indicate that the level of uric acid in the bloodstream of the patient has been a high-level for a number of years. Went to fee is reasonable and apparent and medications and treatment is vital and necessary.

If left alone and untreated for a long period of time gout can lead up to physical deformity and joint damage especially trained physicians will need to employ the most reliable method to diagnose gout. They do this by extracting the fluid from the joint that has been inflamed and they test for the levels of uric acid crystals in order to determine if it is indeed gout.

The extracted fluid is then examined under a microscope in order to find out if uric acid crystals can be found in the specimen. This is an important test to carry out because there are other diseases and medical conditions like pseudogout which is a type of a arthritis brought about by the deposits of calcium Pyrophosphate crystals. The symptoms of pseudogout can have similarities that of gout. It is important for the patient to understand how a change in lifestyle can improve and greatly help in improving their condition and quality of life.

Limiting the consumption of foods mentioned above will not only help in preventing further damage it will also help in avoiding painful flare ups. Treatment and medication for gout typically fall into one of three categories; Prophylactic medications uric acid lowering medications, and rescue medications that give instant relief from the pain caused by gout.

When gout is uncomplicated infrequent and mild the condition can be treated with lifestyle changes and a change of diet. However even the most strict of diets does not decrease the serum uric acid well enough to control and manage severe gout. In this case medications are necessary to treat the condition. Frequent attacks that cost for uric acid kidney stones to occur and the presence of the fee or if joint damage from the gout attacks is evident medications need to be given in order to decrease the uric acid content in the blood level.

Drinking plenty of water for an acute gout attack can be a home remedy. If there are no contraindications such as lowered kidney function or stomach ulcers over-the-counter non - steroidal anti-inflammatory drugs such as ibuprofen and naproxen sodium can be taken by the patient in order to manage the pain. Keeping well hydrated by drinking plenty of water is beneficial to a patient in order to prevent gout attacks.

Chapter Five: Causes of Arthritis

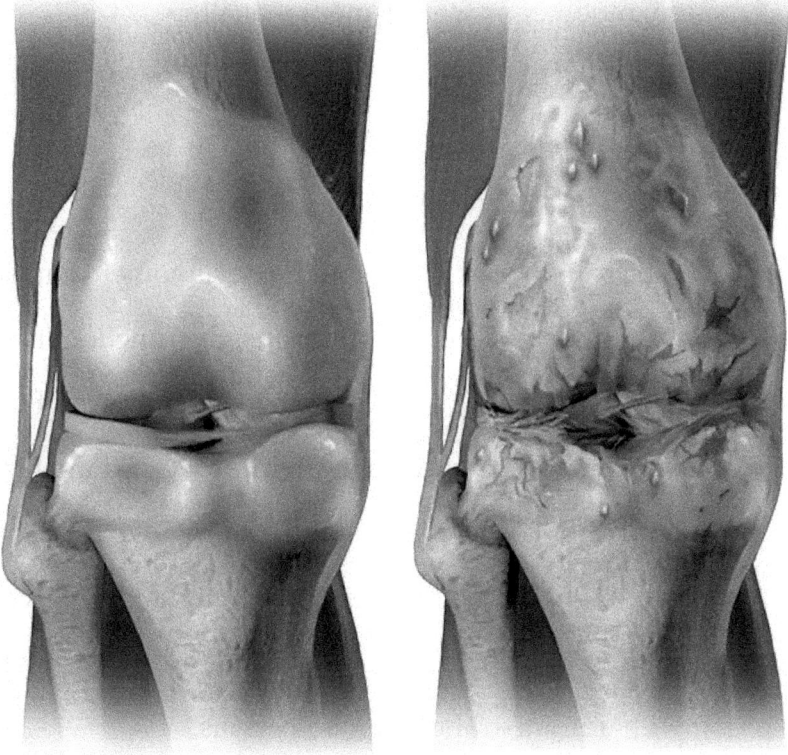

There are about 200 arthritis diseases and conditions which affect the joints and these include osteoarthritis, psoriatic arthritis, gouty arthritis and rheumatoid arthritis. Arthritis can cause a range of indications and symptoms that can inhibit a person's abilities to carry out every day, mundane task. The lack of physical activity can make the condition worse therefore physical activity is recommended to the patient who suffers from arthritis so as to reach the positive results that can help alleviate pain, improve function, mobility as well as mental health.

Factors and Causes

The causes of arthritis and its development can stem from abnormal metabolism, infections, dysfunction in the immune system, past injury or the genetic makeup of the individual. In order to control pain improve and maintain the quality of life of the patient and to minimize damage in the joints, treatment will be needed. Treatment can involve physical therapy, 'patient education, and lifestyle changes along with administration of medications.

Of all the types of arthritis recognized, not one single cause can be pinpointed as the culprit as there are a variety of causes that contribute to the form and sort of arthritis a patient experiences. Some of the causes of arthritis may include abnormal metabolism which can lead to gout or pseudo - gout.

The genetic makeup of a person or a history of arthritis in the family is also another factor that can be the reason of arthritis in an individual. Injuries sustained, whether it is recent or long-standing is also a factor that contributes to the degenerative arthritis of the individual. Lyme disease is one infection that can bring about arthritis. Almost all types of arthritis are associated to have a combination of all these factors. However there are some cases where there are no obvious or apparent reasons and which appear to be unpredictable in its occurrence.

In addition to the causes mentioned above, other reasons linked to the occurrence of arthritis are associated to an infection, physically demanding jobs and smoking. These instances can interact with the patient's genes to further increase their susceptibility and tendency to the risk of arthritis. The diet of a person plays largely in the risk of developing arthritis. Nutrition can also help in managing and avoiding the problems that come along with the occurrence of arthritis in a person.

There are certain foods which provoke a negative response from the immune system which can make the symptoms of arthritis worse by increasing the likelihood of inflammation. Since gout is one sort of arthritis that is closely associated to the diet of a person, unhealthy eating habits can cause the uric acid levels of a person to become elevated.

Who Are the People at Risk?

There are certain risk factors that are linked with arthritis with some being modifiable while others are not. Age is one risk that increases the likelihood of arthritis as a person matures. Another factor contributing to the likelihood of arthritis is the gender of the person. Osteoarthritis is more commonly seen in females, with 60% of arthritis patients being women. On the other hand gout seems to be more common in men than it is in females.

There are specific genes that are linked to certain types of arthritis which elevate the risks of people who have history of the disease in their family. Other contributing factors of people who develop arthritis would be obesity and being overweight. Since excess weight is carried by the joints and bones of the body, the extra pressure put on the joints exacerbates the probability of arthritis developing in a patient. To add to this, there are certain occupations that need to be carried out in a repetitive manner which can lead to the degeneration of protective cartilages.

Infections can also trigger the occurrence of different kinds of arthritis in a person by attacking the joints with microbial agents. Injuries sustained contribute to the development of osteoarthritis. Smoking is another factor that worsens the condition.

Chapter Six: Diagnosing Arthritis

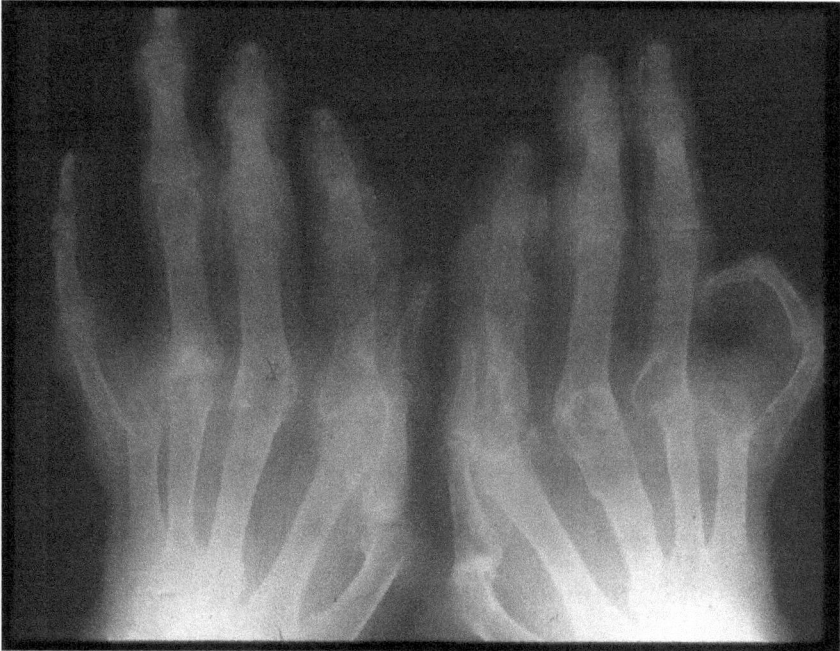

Rheumatoid arthritis is classified as an autoimmune disorder which affects the joints causing chronic inflammation of affected joints of the patient. At the onset of the disorder, mild symptoms that come and go may begin to manifest themselves on either side of the individual's body. This manifestation of chronic inflammation accompanied by pain and difficulty in movement not only develops, it progresses over a period of weeks and months.

The symptoms of the chronic condition are different from one person to the next and even the symptoms a person feels can change from one day to the next. These bouts of symptoms are what are commonly known and called as "flare ups" - when one or more of the symptoms are felt by the individual. When symptoms are absent, this period is known as a remission of the disorder.

Rheumatoid arthritis is one sort of arthritis set of by an affected person's compromised immune system. This is when the immune system zeroes in on the protective lining of affected joints, causing a pronounced amount of pain that was otherwise not present before the development of the disease. RA affects the joints of the hands, wrists, the elbows, feet, ankles and knees of a person. It is also not unusual for the patient suffering from RA to experience pain in the hips. When left untreated, the disease progresses cause a great deal of slow deterioration on the joints and bones of an affected patient.

Along with the damage caused to the vital parts of our joints and bones, which allow us mobility and movement, there are other, various symptoms that manifest it, marking the presence of rheumatoid arthritis in a patient. Rheumatoid arthritis is a chronic condition that has no known cure. Aside from damaging the joints and bones of an individual, it also affects the other systems in the human body. Getting checked as soon as possible is recommended since early detection, diagnosis and treatment increases the chances of being able to reduce the gravity of the symptoms, whilst preventing the condition from getting any worse.

It has been observed and noted that RA is usually identified in adults between the ages of 30 to 50 years old. However, it is not uncommon for it to occur at any age, due to a myriad of reasons. The Arthritis Foundation approximates that there are at least 1.5 million people who have this disease with close to three times that number being women. Although a person who has a family history of RA in their family would have a greater probability of inheriting the disease, people without history of the disease may also develop RA. Patients with RA may not immediately realize that they have the condition and the early onset of the symptoms may go unrecognized, or felt, for years. A person who appears healthy and mobile and active may only realize the condition upon reaching middle age.

How to Recognize the Early Indications and Signs of Rheumatoid Arthritis

Most people with rheumatoid arthritis are diagnosed when they reach middle age, but would have been experiencing the symptoms of the condition long before the actual diagnosis. The symptoms of early rheumatoid arthritis largely go unnoticed because these early episodes happen occasionally and register mild and "insignificant". Other times, the symptoms mimic the symptoms of other conditions, like the flu. Talking about it with a friend who may be going through something similar doesn't help at all, because people don't exhibit the same sort of symptoms.

Symptoms of RA are different in each person, so there is no way to compare or confirm the condition other than going to a physician where one can get a thorough check up and get a proper diagnosis. The experiences of one patient suffering from RA can be totally different from, and not necessarily share the same symptoms with another person suffering from RA.

These symptoms which fluctuate from one to the next sums up three characteristics of the condition; some people only experience the symptoms once and this may not happen again anytime between two to five years making the condition monocyclic. Fluctuating symptoms which seem to worsen then improve, experienced by other patients of the condition is called polycyclic. The third and most common of the characterization of developing rheumatoid arthritis presents itself and progresses to more severe manifestations over time. It does not wane and ebb but is constant. Should any of these symptoms be noticed by an individual, make an appointment with your doctor to determine if the symptoms are indeed RA.

The signs of rheumatoid arthritis can manifest itself in one or more of the following scenarios:

- one or more swollen fingers
- one or more swollen knuckles
- swelling of ankle or knee that last more than 6 weeks
- swelling of elbow or shoulder lasting more than 6 weeks.
- having the sensation of walking on balls
- fever and fatigue
- flu-like symptoms
- tiny, tender bumps beneath the epidermis of the elbow
- stiffness in the joints of the wrists or elbows lasing for an hour or more during the morning.

Early Signs

Symptoms of rheumatoid arthritis can start manifesting itself when a person is around 18 years old, and in most instances, the symptoms are more apparent in the smaller joints of the patient. The joints usually affected are those which connect the fingers to the hands and the feet to the toes. The symptoms are so mild that it is usually ignored and goes unnoticed. The pain that is felt by the patient may come and go; this is called a flare up. Flare ups are set off at certain times then completely fades away at other times. The experience lasts for more than a few days and can even extend for a longer period of time.

These signs include the swelling of the joints, tenderness on the joints when light pressure is applied on the area, feeling a warm sensation in the areas of the joints lasting for more than half an hour during the mornings. Other indications may not be as obvious and may imitate the symptoms for other medical conditions. Some patients develop low grade fever that cannot be explained away.

Then there are those who complain of feeling generally ill without an apparent obvious explanation or cause. There are also patients who experience a loss of appetite during the early stages of rheumatoid arthritis leading to unintended weight loss.

In addition to joint pain and localized tenderness of the area affected, rheumatoid arthritis symptoms become worse as the patient experiences chest pain, labored breathing, as if their breaths are constricted, the patient would also feel numbness and tingling. They experience utterly dry eyes, or in other patients, dry mouth. Patients would also notice red lumps that are painless in the knee region, toes or elbows. Patients may also suffer from anemia.

Chapter Seven: Complications of Arthritis

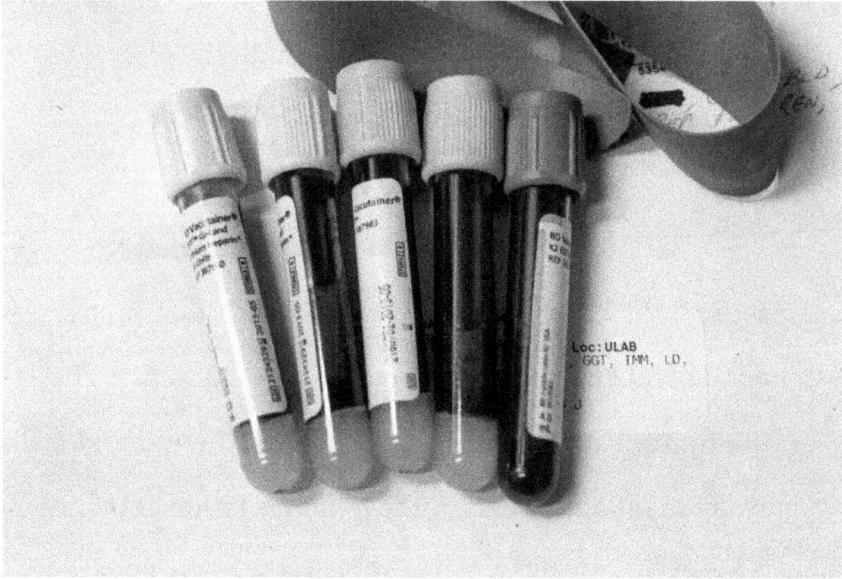

The early symptoms of rheumatoid arthritis include anemia. Anemia is a condition when there is a lack of blood in one's system to supply the rest of the body. This happens when the bone marrow produces a low count of red blood cells than what is actually needed by the body. Red blood cells are responsible for distributing oxygen to the whole body and when fewer red blood cells are in circulation the body essentially lacks the oxygen it needs to operate properly.

Anemia also is the reason why the bone marrow crates lesser hemoglobin, which is the iron-laden protein which transmits vital oxygen to through the blood to the different parts of the body.

Various sorts of anemia are often related to rheumatoid arthritis and these could include iron deficiency anemia and chronic inflammation due to anemia. The autoimmune response of a patient with rheumatoid arthritis results to inflammation of the patient's tissue and joints. When chronic inflammation is active, it causes the bone marrow of the individual to produce lower levels of red blood cells, leading to the production and release of specific proteins which can affect the body in terms of how it uses iron.

Chronic inflammation can also disrupt the manner of how the body manufactures erythropoietin, which is the hormone responsible for and controls the production of red blood cells.

Some medications given to alleviate the pain and discomfort of rheumatoid arthritis like non - steroidal anti - inflammatory medication can lead to the stomach developing bleeding ulcers. Medication such as naproxen, ibuprofen and meloxicam, when taken for prolonged pain management can lead to the digestive tract to bleed. This blood loss becomes a problem that results in the patient to suffer from anemia. If the anemia is too severe, blood transfusions are sometimes necessary to replace the lost blood.

Blood transfusion treatments will help increase not only the red blood cell count it will also elevate the iron levels. Aside from the fact that NSAID drugs causing bleeding in the stomach and digestive tract, these drugs can also cause damage to the liver of the patient. This happens when the food consumed by the individual is stored up and later on released for use. Apart from NSAID medications causing damage to the liver, disease modifying anti - rheumatic drugs, or DMARDs can also result to the same conditions of liver damage and anemia. A patient prescribed

NSAID or DMARDs drugs to manage rheumatoid arthritis will have to undergo routine and intermittent blood tests in order to monitor the presence of anemia.

Anemia in a patient is not only determined through the reports of the patient, but is assisted by thorough check - ups along with vital exams and tests to make sure. A person suffering from anemia would complain of feeling fatigued and weak. They probably have difficulty breathing and would be experiencing shortness of breath. They appear to be pale and they have cold hands and feet. They experience bouts of headaches and chest pains due to the heart getting less oxygenated blood in the supply.

When a person complains of one or more of these conditions, the physician would order the patient to undergo a physical exam to determine if it is indeed anemia the patient is suffering from. It is procedural for the physician to use a stethoscope to listen to the patient's heart and lungs and inspect the abdomen of the patient by pressing on it so that they are able to feel the shape and size of the patient's spleen and liver. Blood tests are ordered by the doctor to make a proper diagnosis and these tests include a red blood cell count, a hemoglobin level exam, a reticulocyte count, a serum ferritin and serum iron. All these tests would determine the measure of new immature blood cells, the protein in the blood as well as the measure of iron in the blood.

Treating Rheumatoid Arthritis Related Anemia

One method in treating RA related anemia is to lessen the inflammation in the body of the patient. Iron supplements are usually given to the patient who has RA related anemia allowing for beneficial iron replacement, however, too much of the iron supplement can also be bad for an individual. Erythropoietin is a drug that can be given to allow for the bone marrow to produce the necessary required red blood cells. It is only given if absolutely necessary to stimulate the production of more red blood cells. The lack of oxygen in the blood results to the heart working overtime and harder to get the proper amount of blood course through the body; therefore it is important that anemia be treated immediately.

The problem of untreated anemia is that the person suffering from it will eventually experience irregular heartbeats, called arrhythmia, and if left this way, this condition could lead to a heart attack. The most commonly seen form of arthritis in people is Osteoarthritis and Rheumatoid Arthritis.

Chapter Eight: Remedies and Treatments

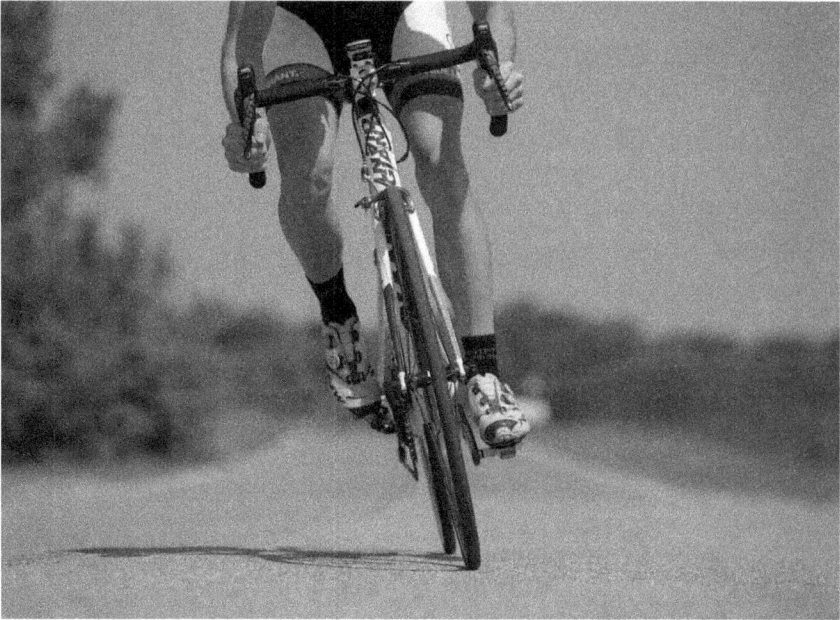

Some people are prone to developing arthritis more than others, and this can depend on a few things like family history, lifestyle and previous injury. Arthritis can change the way the person lives because of the pain that comes along with the condition. Early detection and proper diagnosis are Ways to improve and manage the occurrence and gravity of arthritis. It is important for a person with the disease to understand the importance of switching up the way they eat work and live in order to gain a better handle on the condition.

There are a number of avenues a doctor and patient can take in order to manage the pain of living with arthritis. However it is important that both physician and patient are rigid in following certain treatment options in order for the suffering patient to feel the positive benefits of treatment.

After being given a thorough physical exam which would include blood test, X-rays, MRIs, amongst others, and identifying the sort of arthritis a patient is suffering from, treatment goals are geared toward the pain management of the particular sort of arthritis a patient is experiencing.

Taking Care of Your Joints

Just like the sole of your foot wear, the cartilage which acts as protective portions of the joints in our body also wear away with time. Without the proper protection and padding of the cartilage the bones will end up rubbing against each other which in turn causes massive pain and discomfort. The problem with a worn out cartilage is that once it is frayed it does not here nor does it grow back.

And this is my arthritis is said to be a condition that has no known cure. Once it begins it is only a matter of time until degeneration takes place, therefore it is very important to realize how vital the function of the cartilage is to our joints and overall well-being. Knowing what steps to take in order to lead a better quality of life has to be undertaken by the patient and followed in order to alleviate pain and suffering caused by arthritis.

Medications

Over-the-counter painkillers can help manage the pain brought about by ice right this for short periods of time especially during flare ups. Some of the more common Pain relievers are ibuprofen, acetaminophen and Naproxen. These are good choices for short-term relief from arthritis pain however you should always consult with your doctor about the amount of pain relievers that you take and how often you should take them. Should you be taking them for a long period of time it may be necessary to talk about joint replacement surgery. You may also discuss Cortisone shots that could be helpful for short term flare ups.

Gout medications are recommended when it is tolerated by the individual however like most other medications in the market that is given to patients these drugs have potential side effects. Side effects may include allergic rash symptoms such as diarrhea and nausea as well as abnormal blood counts and muscle weakness. Some medications can exacerbate and worsen the kidney stones while others can cause irritation of the stomach lining and develop ulcers in some patients.

Therapy

Stretching is a good way to keep a person, suffering from arthritis, flexible. Now only does it why flexible it also improves the patient's range of motion and the way you can move your joints. This also is beneficial because it helps the patient decreased the odds of injuries and pain caused by arthritis.

Make sure that you always start your exercises and workouts with a five minute warm-up walk. After this you may lie on your back and stretch your hamstrings by looping a bitch around your phone using the sheet to help pull the leg straight up in the air. Hold this for at least 20 seconds then lower the leg you should take this twice on both legs.

You may want to consider the traditional Chinese medicine of acupuncture which involves insertion of find needles to certain target points on the body which can help alleviate pain and manage it.

Exercise

Make it a point to shed pounds if you are overweight or obese. The extra weight that we carry puts a lot of pressure on the joints and on the protective cartilage that acts as padding between the joints. Losing weight will help take away the stress from your hips and knees. Every pound lost removes 4 pounds of pressure that is put on the knees that affects the patient.

Losing weight lessons the wear and tear in the joint and may actually slow the progress of arthritis. For every 10 pounds that is lost relief is felt because it will reduce the pain by at least 20%. Exercising is important in order to slow down the deterioration that is happening within the body and causing the pain of arthritis. The pain it still may make the individual hesitant to exercise and workout. But research has shown and proven that the stiffness and pain caused by arthritis only gets worse when a person is inactive.

Exercising regularly will get the heart pumping and will increase the blood flow in the body. Increased blood flow allows the cartilage to stay well - nourished and function properly. And as an extra benefit exercising helps the individual attain a healthy weight in order to keep in shape and manage the pain of arthritis. Staying as active as possible is very important make sure that your activity is something that is suited for you and approved by your doctor.

Avoid high impact activities such as running and jumping. It is best to choose exercises that are low impact like brisk walking cycling and swimming.

Possessing muscles that are strong around the joints can help the body take in some of the names that normally courses through the joint when in movement. Strong muscles have ability to absorb the shock that is normally felt by the joints. Ask your doctor or physical therapist what sort of workout you can do in order to build up the muscles that surround your joints doing so will improve the symptoms in your name and ankles. Only work with a personal trainer or physical therapist that has experience working with people who have arthritis.

Make it a point to stretch every day; stretching your body will help improve your mobility and your ability to move your joints without too much pain. Stretching not only towards of stiffness but it also assist in the protection of the cartilage from the normal wear and tear up every day activities. Some doctors recommend that their patience to

Pilates or yoga in order for their patience to be more flexible. There is no need to attempt to be an expert in your yoga or Pilates classes,

The Dos and Don'ts of Knee Pain

Whether you have sustained an injury from a recent accident or if you are suffering from any pain due to arthritis there are certain things that you should remember to avoid and so as not to encourage their albums or further the injury. There are also a few things that you should remember to do in order to manage your pain.

Continue with activity that you can tolerate and exercise as we quickly as you can. Cardio exercises are suggested in order to strengthen the muscles that carry the weight of your knees. Cardio exercises not only strengthen the muscles allowing for more confident movement it also increases your flexibility. In addition to these stretching, it's also very important to strengthen the muscles that surround the joints will not only allow you better mobility it will also curb the massive pain that patients who have arthritis endure.

When you experience any knee pain from an arthritis flare up or one that is caused by an injury, remember to give yourself a rest. You should then apply ice to the affected area so as to reduce swelling and inflammation. To prevent further pain, use a compression bandage and elevate the leg in order to recover from the flare up; if absolutely needed do not hesitate to use a cane, a crutch or a walking aid to take some of the stress off of the knee when in motion.

Aside from walking aids people with arthritis can also utilize braces and splints to keep their balance while walking or when standing. When the knee is unstable or in pain, there is a higher likelihood for the person to fall and cause more damage to the knee area. Avoid these risks of falling by ensuring that your home is equipped with handrails on staircases. If you need to reach for something that is situated at a high-level it is best to use a sturdy ladder or a footstool to help you do the job.

Be sure to be mindful of your footwear as it can make matters worse. If you have osteoarthritis or any sorts of arthritis for that matter make sure that you use cushioned insoles so that it reduces the stress on your ball joints knees and hips.

A woman separate from any form of arthritis should try to avoid using high heels as these can exacerbate the condition. So best to find the proper insole for your footwear it is advise that you speak to a physical therapist or your specialist about what sort of insoles they recommend.

In the event of an injury use of cold pack to Isa swelling and to numb the pain of the injured area. You may utilize a frozen bag of peas or a bag filled with ice. apply the, wrapped in soft cloth, ice pack to the localized affected area for about fifteen to twenty minutes three to four times each day. Switch it out by taking a warm bath or applying a warm towel or heating pad to the area for about 15 to 20 minutes as well 3 to 4 times daily in essence you want to alternate cold and hot compresses in order to ease the swelling.

Your doctor therapist and physical trainer will advise you against taking up any high impact exercises which can ensure you further and cause worst damage and pain. Jarring exercises including kickboxing, jumping rope, leaping from a high place, running, Lunges and deep squats are high impact exercises that create a lot of stress and put a lot of pressure on an individual's knees. Not only do these high impact exercises cause more stress to the knees were sent to pain it can also cause further injury.

The symptoms of arthritis are different in one person to the next. Each individual go through a variety of indications and symptoms that is not necessarily experienced by other arthritic patients. Therefore it is absolutely imperative that you had out and see a doctor in order to get properly tested and diagnosed. This will enable the doctor the recommend the proper medicine the correct exercise and any other walking aids that may be beneficial and helpful to the patient.

Replacement Surgery

If you have been taking anti-inflammatory medications and pain relievers for an extended period of time it may be wise to talk to your doctor about joint replacement surgery. The problem with prolonged use of anti-inflammatory drugs is that these medications can take a toll on your liver. If you have been kind to your knees by giving it a rest, if you have utilized the aid of a cane, brace or splint, if you gave physical therapy a fair chance, if you have followed doctor's orders and lost the pounds, and still experience frequent discomfort and difficulty in movement, you may have to consider surgery.

If you still experience a lot of pain and difficulty getting out of bed in the morning or if your knee remains swollen and has started to bow, the symptoms may indicate that you may possibly need knee replacement surgery.

Although the most typically replaced joint in the body is the need this does not mean that your orthopedic surgeon will make this decision for you on the whim.

Knee replacement surgery is not taken lightly and the process begins with the doctor determining the medical history of the patient making sure to know they have the information about your general health and the specifics of the pain you experience on the me and most especially how arthritis affects your quality of life.

Your doctor will recommend tests in order to find out the alignment of your leg the stability, strength and motion of your knees. An X-ray will give the surgeon a better inside of whether the bone is deformed or damaged. And accompanying MRI gives the surgeon a more detailed look into the soft tissues surrounding your knee and a deeper look into the bone and cartilage itself. Blood tests and laboratory exams are possible procedures that a patient of arthritis will have to undergo in order to rule out or identify other reasons and causes for the pain experienced in the knees.

Should the physician decide to proceed with the total knee replacement he will be given detailed information about the possible problems and risks that entail the surgery. You will also be given information on what to expect after surgery and what you need to do in order to maintain the knee replacement. The first order of business that the doctor will discuss with the patient would be to lose any extra poundage that the patient may be carrying to alleviate some of the stress that is being experienced by the knees.

A Change in Diet and Eating Habits

Aside from giving advice to lose weight doctors will also investigate what sort of food a patient with rightists usually has. Diet plays a big factor in the development of arthritis in persons between the ages of 30 to 50 years old. Therefore indulging in foods that promote arthritis will need to be avoided in order to see the positive results of the treatment. Since gout is commonly linked with obesity, significant weight loss can improve the management of the condition dramatically. Reducing calorie intake is a good way to shed pounds.

Doctors would usually recommend a diet that is low in saturated fat. They would normally recommend the replacement of refined carbohydrates like white bread potatoes and sugar with complex carbohydrates like whole grains and vegetables which help reduce the serum uric acid.

The doctor will strongly advise the patient to avoid frequent consumption of red meat and seafood. Avoidance of liquor and beer consumption will also be strongly recommended by the physician since alcoholic beverages increase the risk of gout. Aside from alcoholic beverages increasing the risk of a gallon sweetened beverages that is high in fructose corn syrup also heightens the possibility of the development of gout. And because that is a chronic condition if left untreated the patient may experience repeated painful and immobilizing acute flare ups of gout.

Complications of doubt may develop if it is not treated and eventual joint damage will be a parent and leave the patient immobilized with their quality of life compromised. Some of the risk factors of gout is hereditary and genetic and these make a predisposition for gout and preventable. However other risk factors can be curbed, like obesity diet and lifestyle.

Chapter Nine: Alternative Pain Management

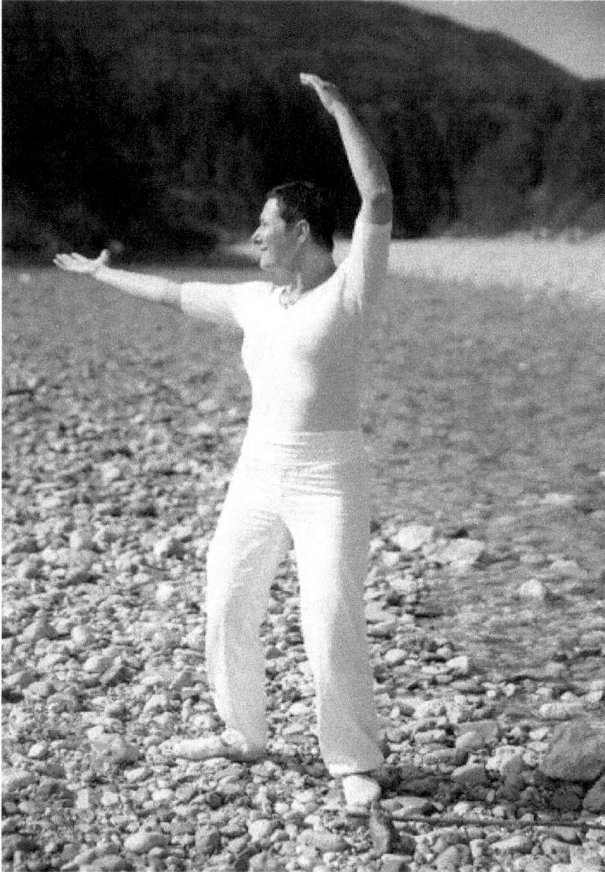

No matter how a patient ends up developing any form of arthritis, whether from injury or the extra poundage that puts pressure on the joints, or genetically passed on, all results are pretty much similar and unmistakable- pain and compromised movement as well as limited mobility and a shift in the quality of life are all some of the commonalities of arthritis in all patients. It is important that the patient experiencing pain due to arthritis, see a doctor and get tested and properly diagnosed to get the proper treatment that they need.

If you are looking for ways to ease the pain and delay or avoid undergoing knee replacement surgery read up and find out about what you can do alternatively to taking over-the-counter or prescribed medication. The most common recommendation and medical advice that physicians would give patients who have osteoarthritis or rheumatoid arthritis are to exercise. Inactivity does not help curb the pain that is brought about by arthritis. In fact extended or prolonged periods of rest can in fact make the condition worse and lead to depression due to the change experience by the individual.

Shed Those Extra Pounds

Shedding extra weight is a heavy emphasis that doctors strongly suggest to their patients because regular exercise is one of the best way to not only get relief from the pain caused by arthritis it is also beneficial in terms of keeping the weight of the patient at bay so as not to put any more added pressure on the affected joints.

Building and strengthening the muscles that surround the joints is also another method that works positively toward relieving and curbing the pain brought about by arthritis. Shedding even just a fraction of the way it shows in Normas positive if X because each pound that is shed lessons the weight on the joints by 4 pounds. Shedding just 5% of the body weight increases the patient's ability to move and makes a big impact on the reduction of pain.

Losing a more significant amount slows the process of the disease and this has shown positive effects and a better quality of life in the patients who have heeded to this medical advice. Physical exercise not only makes it easier for the person to lose weight it also allows the person to maintain a proper weight that is not a deterrent to their condition. The lack of exercise causes a domino effect due to the inactivity of the individual which can lead to weakened muscles increased pain less mobility and the worsening of the condition.

Physicians would typically recommend that you exercise so it is best to find an experienced physical trainer or Hera pissed who can give you the best advice on what sort of exercises is good for you. Patients with arthritis are discouraged from taking part in rigorous high impact physical activity and are advised to take up low impact exercises, like yoga, tai-chi, Pilates.

Tai Chi

Tai Chi is a low impact exercise with flowing movements done in a slow fashion and is recommended by many doctors since it helps in the pain management and physical function by up to about 35%. Tai Chi is a low impact exercise with flowing movements done in a slow fashion and is recommended by many doctors since it helps in the pain management and physical function by up to about 35%. Since arthritis is a mind body disease you will need to combat this with the mind body exercise like Tai Chi which not only helps to keep the patient flexible active while managing the pain it also lowers stress in patients.

Work with Your Physical Therapist

With the help of a physical therapist you can work on targeting the weak spots that has been bothersome and painful and importantly can improve not only the balance but also the strength and joint alignment of the patient. Since arthritis has no known cure yet constant research is being done in order to provide more detailed guidance on how to treat people with arthritis. And arthritis patient has to take the responsibility of understanding their condition in order to avoid events that may cause further damage to their joints and most especially the cartilage.

Making it a point to build a strong understanding of how arthritis affects the body and the options available in terms of treatment and therapy is the best strategy for coping and managing arthritis. Learn more about the disease including things that you need to avoid doing so as not to worsen the condition.

Self – Management and Discipline

Self-management and discipline is very important if you want to improve your deteriorated quality of life. Many people who suffer from arthritis are afraid to exercise because they think that putting added weight on their joints will worsen the condition when in fact knowing the rights of exercise that will help you will not only assist in slowing down the progress of the disease it will also give you a better mental outlook of positivity towards managing the disease.

You want to know what you are up against so that you know what to do and what to avoid. Some exercises can in fact cause more stress and more damage to the joints like the rapid pivoting moves during a football game or the movements carried out when skateboarding or downhill skiing. Understanding your physical limitations and sticking to a low impact program will greatly help you in managing the condition without furthering the damage to the joints. Do not attend exercise immediately if you have not at least warmed up for five minutes by way of stretching.

Acupuncture

Although there is little recorded medical evidence that acupuncture is beneficial many patients who have done for these procedures has shown some sort of benefit interims of patients who have multiple health problems that inhibit them from other treatment options. Ask your doctor about acupuncture and get their approval if you would like to try the procedure and see if it does in fact have any benefit to your condition. Make sure that you ask your doctor for a recommendation or look for an accredited acupuncturist practitioner who can help you with your expertise.

Balneotherapy or Spa Therapy

There have been recent studies on the benefits of Balneotherapy or spa therapy. Spa therapy includes soaking the affected area in heated mineral water or soaking in mud baths or a water massage. New studies support water therapy in the improvement and management of arthritis pain. Spa therapy is usually recommended to patients who have some creating conditions and multiple joint damage that have restrictions and limitations in the treatment options available to them.

Research is showing that water therapy help in improving stiffness and pain in some patients who go for a procedure for an hour a day for at least three weeks. Balneotherapy is more common in Europe then it is in the states however if you ask your doctor your physician specialist may be able to suggest similar facilities that provide similar treatments.

Biomechanics and Therapeutic Equipment

The alignment of hips knees spine and feet is important to the wellness of a person. When issues with biomechanics arise this worsens pain felt by the patient. Joint alignment devices have many types and a lot of them can either be off the shelf biomechanical devices or custom built biomechanical devices which could include various types of braces, therapeutic shoes, including wedged insoles. Ask your specialist about biomechanical devices or get a biomechanical evaluation from the proper specialist or physical therapist to get the best device to help you. These tools and devices when worn by people with arthritis such as knee braces or foot orthotics help lessen the pain and decrease joint stiffness. The use of these devices may also help in lessening pain medication intake.

Herbal Remedies

More and more patients who have arthritis are looking to botanicals and herbs to help manage the symptoms of arthritis. Although medicine and medications have changed the way in treating disorders such as this more and more patients who have arthritis are looking to botanicals and herbs to help manage the symptoms of arthritis. Many patients have chosen to explore another avenue of pain management through substances derived from plants.

Consumer reports in the United States state that more than half of adults in the United States take botanicals and other natural remedies to prevent or treat disease. It is an industry that takes in about $30 billion each year. A majority of the people included in that demographic our patients who suffer from arthritis. As with any other treatment for whatever condition it is strongly advise that you consult with your doctor before taking any herbal remedies. And because arthritis is a disease that causes inflammation and joint distraction as well as organ damage patients are never advised to rely on herbal remedies alone.

Make sure that you consult with your doctor before you take any of the supplements in order for you to fully be aware of any potential interactions to the medication prescribed to you and the possible side effects.

Botanicals come in many forms and in different varieties. The studies conducted on botanicals are commonly compared to standardize extracts that can be found in the form of pills there for utilizing other sorts may make it difficult The exact the proper amount as well as the active ingredient that the patient will be getting consult with your doctor and find an herbal specialist who has a track record of success in the field of botanical medicine.

Herbal remedies can be taken in infusions by adding the plant or herb to boiling water. These herbal remedies and botanicals could be in the form of flowers leaves, stems or roots. Some plants May only require just a few minutes of stepping in water whereas other plant products we require a longer amount of time for the active components to be released.

The most popular sort of botanicals sold is tea and it is one of the most well-known forms of herbal remedies. Tea is made through a process of infusion by adding boiling water dried plant products or fresh leaves roots stems are flowers. It requires just a few minutes of steeping. Mixture of herbal components and ingredients is called a concoction and can be prepared in several ways. It is usually prepared with heat. The process of adding a variety of plant products to boiling water like roots, berries or bark, is called decoction. When the preparation is complete the liquid derived from the decoction is drunk.

Liquid forms of botanical medicine, such as extract-drinks and oils are preparations made with water and alcohol. These are called tinctures. These extracts are created equal using a variety of solvents and liquids where in the liquid is allowed to evaporate in order to draw out a dry extract. Once the dry extracts are complete they are formed into tablets or placed inside capsules and packaged. Extract and tincture are more concentrated than herbs produced as tea. Lastly dried or fresh herbs are ingredients that can be grown or purchased.

Herb and Supplement Guide

- Black currant oil
- Boswellia
- Capsaicin
- Chondroitin sulfate
- Devils claw
- Dimethyl sulfoxide
- Fish oil
- Ginger
- Gamma-linolenic acid
- Green-lipped mussel
- Melatonin
- Pine bark
- Sam-E
- Stinging nettle
- Turmeric
- Valerian

- Thunder god vine

- St. John's wort

- Rose hips

- MSM

- Melatonin

- Indian frankincense

- Green lipped mussel

- Glucosamine

- Ginkgo

- Flaxseed

- Evening primrose

- DHEA

- curcumin

- Cat's claw

- Avocado soybean unsaponifiables

Chapter Ten: Summary

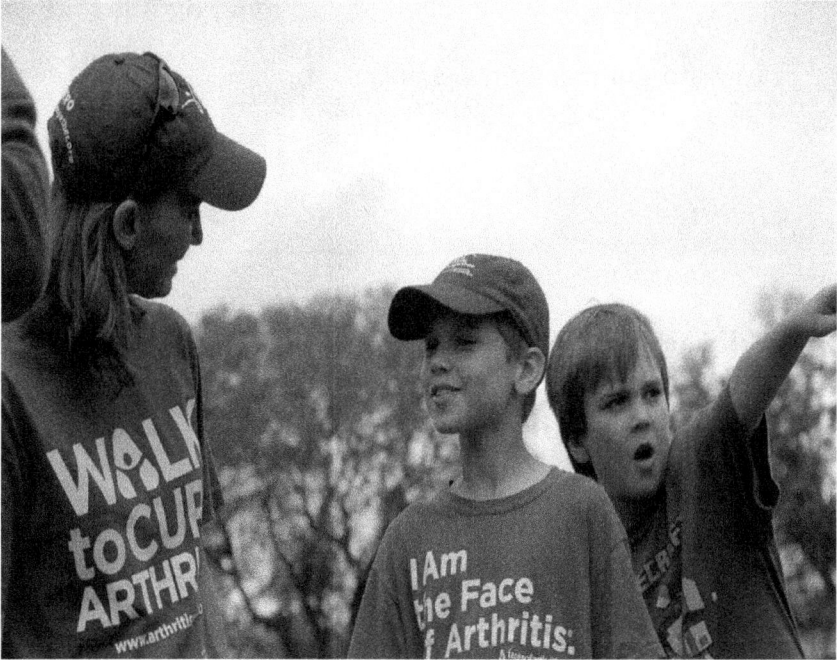

Knowing the symptoms of arthritis can greatly help in arresting whatever damage is being caused to the cardiologist and bones of the individual. Recognizing the signs and indications that point to arthritis can power an individual to get help from a doctor to get proper diagnosis in order to find the best possible treatment for the sort of arthritis they suffer from. Apart from going to a doctor getting all the possible tests and getting the proper diagnosis it is the responsibility of the individual suffering from arthritis to understand the disease so that they are better able systems live a lifestyle that makes it possible for them to carry out your daily tasks and routine.

Highlights

Risk Factors of Arthritis

Abnormal Metabolism: When a person's metabolism is out of whack, the anomaly can lead to gout or pseudo - gout.

Degenerative Arthritis: This is stem out from an injury sustained which could develop into more severe complications.

Lyme Disease: A disease born of a tick bite is also a cause for painful arthritis in a patient

Symptoms of Arthritis

Fatigue: The body responds to the effects of the disease resulting in poor sleep quality brought about by pain. Fatigue is the body's way of reacting to the inflammation experienced by the patient's joints. It can also be brought about by the body's reaction to medication.

Joint Pains: It is not unusual for inflammation to also take place should the joints already have suffered previous damage. When rheumatoid arthritis is active, it paves the way for the joints to swell up because of the lining tissue of the joint thickening and also to the excess joint fluid present in the localized area. When this transpires, the swollen joint expands and stretches out, irritating the capsule that encloses the joint.

Tenderness and Loss of Range of Motion: Movement is not only limited because of the pain it is constrained as well because of the amount of pain and discomfort. This is why people suffering from RA often, at the very least suffer from interrupted sleep and at its extreme, insomnia.

Swelling and Stiffness: Stiffness of the joints or difficulty in mobility and movement is another symptom of RA. This is when the joints affected by active RA are swollen and stiff. Stiffness of the joint is usually more apparent and felt in the morning rather than any other time of the day.

Redness and Warmth: The capillaries of the skin over the inflamed region widens due to the nearby inflamed joints of the area. The widened capillaries, also called dilated capillaries exacerbate the situation and display it apparent. When the affected joints of the patient are inflamed and the RA is active, the joints are warm to the touch. When this happens the affected areas become swollen, tender, warm and painful.

Deformity of Joints: When left unchecked and untreated, inflammation of the areas affected leads up to the deterioration of the cartilage and bone whilst loosening the ligament of the affected region. When left unchecked, permanent joint deformity and ruin will occur.

Limping: Limping could be caused by a number of other ailments of the muscles, bones and nerves; a noticeable limp exhibited by the individual is caused by extreme pain and discomfort, a loss of range of motion of the affected areas, and is accompanied by swelling of the joint.

Common Forms of Arthritis

Rheumatoid Arthritis

- This form of arthritis is classified as an autoimmune disease wherein the immune system of the individual suffering from the disease attacks parts of the body.

- When the immune systems attacks the joints, the affected joints of the patient become swollen and this can eventually lead to damage of the joints if left untreated.

Symptoms:

- Patients usually complain of stiffness and pain, reporting the sensation of their joints feeling "fused" together.

- The stiffness, swelling and pain is usually felt in the wrists and/or hands, the elbows and/or shoulders, the knees and/or ankles, the feet, jaw and/or neck of the patient.

Osteoarthritis

- Osteoarthritis happens when the cartilage that protects and covers the ends of the bones erode and wear down over time.

- This condition can be present anywhere in the patient's body but is most commonly seen affecting the joints of the hands, knees, hips and spine.

Symptoms:

- The symptoms of this ailment can typically be managed effectively through treatment, therapy and medication (or the combination of two or all methods of management) but the process, once it has begun, is usually irreversible.

- Physical indications of osteoarthritis include pain in the joints while in motion or after movement.

- Tenderness of the joint affected is apparent when light pressure is applied to the area in question.

- Stiffness of the joint is most apparent upon waking in the morning; stiffness may also be apparent to the patient suffering from the disease after a period of inactivity.

- The loss of flexibility on the affected area is seen, and the full range of motion is depleted.

- Bone spurs, or extra bone bits that form around the affected joints, feel like hard lumps.

Psoriatic Arthritis

- The condition typically targets individuals between the ages of 30 to 50 years of age. Psoriatic arthritis is a rare disease as it is utterly damaging.

- The destruction caused by this form of arthritis quickly damages the joints of the patient at the tips of their toes and fingers rendering them useless.

- The tendons of the psoriatic arthritis patient could also become affected through time.

Symptoms:

- It typically manifests itself through the joints causing them to swell. The joints would then get very painful and puffed up. The affected joints would feel hot to the touch and looks like angry red welts. The fingers and toes of a patient affected with psoriatic arthritis would puff up and look like swollen sausages.

- Stiffness and pain in the neck, the upper and lower back, as well as the buttocks may stem from the swelling in the joints of the spine and the hip bones of the patient, making movement and mobility painful and limited.

- Tiny dents and ridges, called pitting, are apparent on the nails of both hands and feet of the patient with psoriatic arthritis

- The eyes too can become affected, making the colored portion of the eye

- Shortness of breath accompanied by chest pains can be some of the symptoms a patient with psoriatic arthritis experiences.

- Psoriatic arthritis can also manifest itself through red, itchy blotches on the skin. It also manifest on the skin as thick, gray, scale like protrusions

Gout

- Gout is a sort of arthritis which results in a sudden swelling of affected joints. This condition is developed by uric acid crystals being deposited in the affected joint and can cause symptoms such as the appearance of nodules beneath the skin (tophi).

Symptoms:

- The signs and symptoms of gout typically affect one joint; the pain that the patient feels is usually very severe and is reflective of the seriousness of the swelling in the joint. The affected area is tender and warm to the touch and there are some instances when even the slightest movement or brushing of object against it causes excruciating pain.

- Gout usually affects the joints of the lower extremities of the patient's body usually are getting the big toe.

- Gout can also be recognized through the presence of tophi. This is a hard nodule of uric acid that is concentrated under the localized affected area of the skin.

Causes of Arthritis

- The causes of arthritis and its development can stem from abnormal metabolism, infections, dysfunction in the immune system, past injury or the genetic makeup of the individual.

- Some of the causes of arthritis may include abnormal metabolism which can lead to gout or pseudo - gout.

- The genetic makeup of a person or a history of arthritis in the family is also another factor that can be the reason of arthritis in an individual.

- Injuries sustained, whether it is recent or long-standing is also a factor that contributes to the degenerative arthritis of the individual.

- Other reasons linked to the occurrence of arthritis are associated to an infection, physically demanding jobs and smoking. These instances can interact with the patient's genes to further increase their susceptibility and tendency to the risk of arthritis.

- There are certain foods which provoke a negative response from the immune system which can make the symptoms of arthritis worse by increasing the likelihood of inflammation.

Who Are the People at Risk?

- Age is one risk that increases the likelihood of arthritis as a person matures. Another factor contributing to the likelihood of arthritis is the gender of the person.

- Another factor contributing to the likelihood of arthritis is the gender of the person; 60% of arthritis patients being women

- There are specific genes that are linked to certain types of arthritis which elevate the risks of people who have history of the disease in their family.

- Other contributing factors of people who develop arthritis would be obesity and being overweight. Since excess weight is carried by the joints and bones of the body, the extra pressure put on the joints exacerbates the probability of arthritis developing in a patient.

- Infections can also trigger the occurrence of different kinds of arthritis in a person by attacking the joints with microbial agents

Diagnosing Arthritis

- Most people with rheumatoid arthritis are diagnosed when they reach middle age, but would have been experiencing the symptoms of the condition long before the actual diagnosis.

- The symptoms mimic the symptoms of other conditions like the flu

- Symptoms which fluctuate from one to the next sums up three characteristics of the condition; some people only experience the symptoms once and this may not happen again anytime between two to five years making the condition monocyclic.

- Fluctuating symptoms which seem to worsen then improve, experienced by other patients of the condition is called polycyclic.

The signs of rheumatoid arthritis can manifest itself in one or more of the following scenarios:

- One or more swollen fingers
- One or more swollen knuckles
- Swelling of ankle or knee that last more than 6 weeks

- Swelling of elbow or shoulder lasting more than 6 weeks.

- Having the sensation of walking on balls

- Fever and fatigue

- Flu-like symptoms

- Tiny, tender bumps beneath the epidermis of the elbow

- Stiffness in the joints of the wrists or elbows lasing for an hour or more during the morning.

Complications of Arthritis

Anemia and Arthritis

- Anemia is the reason why the bone marrow crates lesser hemoglobin, which is the iron-laden protein which transmits vital oxygen to through the blood to the different parts of the body.

- Various sorts of anemia are often related to rheumatoid arthritis and these could include iron deficiency anemia and chronic inflammation due to anemia.

- The autoimmune response of a patient with rheumatoid arthritis results to inflammation of the patient's tissue and joints.

- Chronic inflammation can also disrupt the manner of how the body manufactures erythropoietin, which is the hormone responsible for and controls the production of red blood cells.

Treating Rheumatoid Arthritis Related Anemia

- One method in treating RA related anemia is to lessen the inflammation in the body of the patient. Iron supplements are usually given to the patient who has RA related anemia allowing for beneficial iron replacement.

- Erythropoietin is a drug that can be given to allow for the bone marrow to produce the necessary required red blood cells. It is only given if absolutely necessary to stimulate the production of more red blood cells.

- The problem of untreated anemia is that the person suffering from it will eventually experience irregular heartbeats, called arrhythmia, and if left this way, this condition could lead to a heart attack.

Remedies and Treatments

Take Care of Your Joints

- The cartilage which acts as protective portions of the joints in our body wears out over time. Without the proper protection and padding of the cartilage the bones will end up rubbing against each other which in turn causes massive pain and discomfort.

- Once it begins it is only a matter of time until degeneration takes place, therefore it is very important to realize how vital the function of the cartilage is to our joints and overall well-being

Medications

- Some of the more common Pain relievers are ibuprofen, acetaminophen and Naproxen. These are good choices for short-term relief from arthritis pain however you should always consult with your doctor about the amount of pain relievers that you take and how often you should take them.

- Gout medications are recommended when it is tolerated by the individual however like most other medications in the market that is given to patients these drugs have potential side effects.

Exercise

- Make sure that you always start your exercises and workouts with a five minute warm-up walk. After this you may lie on your back and stretch your hamstrings by looping a bitch around your phone using the sheet to help pull the leg straight up in the air.

- Hold this for at least 20 seconds then lower the leg you should take this twice on both legs.

- Strong muscles have ability to absorb the shock that is normally felt by the joints. Ask your doctor or physical therapist what sort of workout you can do in order to build up the muscles that surround your joints.

Replacement Surgery

- If you have been taking anti-inflammatory medications and pain relievers for an extended period of time it may be wise to talk to your doctor about joint replacement surgery.

- Your doctor will recommend tests in order to find out the alignment of your leg the stability, strength and motion of your knees.

- An X-ray will give the surgeon a better inside of whether the bone is deformed or damaged.

- MRI gives the surgeon a more detailed look into the soft tissues surrounding your knee and a deeper look into the bone and cartilage itself.

- Blood tests and laboratory exams are possible procedures that a patient of arthritis will have to undergo in order to rule out or identify other reasons and causes for the pain experienced in the knees.

Change in Diet and Eating Habits

- Doctors would usually recommend a diet that is low in saturated fat. They would normally recommend the replacement of refined carbohydrates like white bread potatoes and sugar with complex carbohydrates like whole grains and vegetables which help reduce the serum uric acid.

- Avoidance of liquor and beer consumption will also be strongly recommended by the physician since alcoholic beverages increase the risk of gout.

- The doctor will strongly advise the patient to avoid frequent consumption of red meat and seafood

Alternative Pain Management

Shed Those Extra Pounds

- Losing a more significant amount slows the process of the disease and this has shown positive effects and a better quality of life in the patients who have heeded to this medical advice.

- Physical exercise not only makes it easier for the person to lose weight it also allows the person to maintain a proper weight that is not a deterrent to their condition.

- Patients with arthritis are discouraged from taking part in rigorous high impact physical activity and are advised to take up low impact exercises, like yoga and Tai-chi.

Tai Chi

- Tai Chi is a low impact exercise with flowing movements done in a slow fashion and is recommended by many doctors since it helps in the pain management and physical function by up to about 35%

Work with Your Physical Therapist

- Making it a point to build a strong understanding of how arthritis affects the body and the options available in terms of treatment and therapy is the best strategy for coping and managing arthritis.

Self – Management and Discipline

- Understanding your physical limitations and sticking to a low impact program will greatly help you in managing the condition without furthering the damage to the joints.

- Do not attend exercise immediately if you have not at least warmed up for five minutes by way of stretching.

Acupuncture

- Ask your doctor about acupuncture and get their approval if you would like to try the procedure and see if it does in fact have any benefit to your condition.

- Make sure that you ask your doctor for a recommendation or look for an accredited acupuncturist practitioner who can help you with your expertise.

Balneotherapy or Spa Therapy

- Spa therapy includes soaking the affected area in heated mineral water or soaking in mud baths or a water massage

- Research is showing that water therapy help in improving stiffness and pain in some patients who go for a procedure for an hour a day for at least three weeks

- Balneotherapy is more common in Europe then it is in the states however if you ask your doctor your physician specialist may be able to suggest similar facilities that provide similar treatments

Biomechanics

- Ask your specialist about biomechanical devices or get a biomechanical evaluation from the proper specialist or physical therapist to get the best device to help you

- These tools and devices when worn by people with arthritis such as knee braces or foot orthotics help lessen the pain and decrease joint stiffness

Herbal Remedies

- Herbal remedies can be taken in infusions by adding the plant or herb to boiling water. These herbal remedies and botanicals could be in the form of flowers leaves, stems or roots.

- Some plants May only require just a few minutes of stepping in water whereas other plant products we require a longer amount of time for the active components to be released

- The most popular sort of botanicals sold is tea and it is one of the most well-known forms of herbal remedies.

- Tinctures are liquid forms of botanical medicine, such as extract-drinks and oils are preparations made with water and alcohol.

Photo Credits

References

15 Early Symptoms and Signs of Rheumatoid Arthritis (RA) – MedicineNet.com

https://www.medicinenet.com/rheumatoid_arthritis_early_symptoms/article.htm

About Arthritis – Arthritis.org

https://www.arthritis.org

Diagnosing Arthritis – Arthritis.org

https://www.arthritis.org/about-arthritis/understanding-arthritis/diagnosing-arthritis.php

How is RA-related anemia treated? – HealthLine.com

https://www.healthline.com/health/rheumatoid-arthritis-and-anemia#treatment

Inflammation and Arthritis – WebMD.com

https://www.webmd.com/arthritis/arthritis-inflammation#1

Juvenile Idiopathic Arthritis (JIA, Arthritis in Childhood, Juvenile Rheumatoid Arthritis, JRA, Juvenile Chronic Arthritis) – MedicineNet.com

https://www.medicinenet.com/juvenile_arthritis/article.htm

Osteoarthritis – Mayoclinic.org

https://www.mayoclinic.org/diseases-
conditions/osteoarthritis/diagnosis-treatment/drc-20351930

Psoriatic Arthritis Tests and Diagnosis – WebMD.com

https://www.webmd.com/arthritis/psoriatic-
arthritis/psoriatic-arthritis-diagnosis

Sources of Arthritis Pain – Arthritis.org

https://www.arthritis.org/living-with-arthritis/pain-
management/understanding/types-of-pain.php

Top 3 Types of Arthritis – WebMD.com

https://www.webmd.com/rheumatoid-arthritis/guide/most-
common-arthritis-types#1

Understanding Arthritis -- Diagnosis & Treatment –
WebMD.com

https://www.webmd.com/arthritis/understanding-arthritis-
treatment#1

What Type of Arthritis Do You Have? – HealthLine.com

https://www.healthline.com/health/arthritis-types

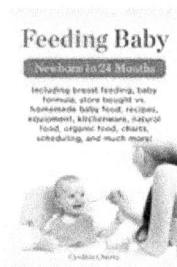

Feeding Baby
Cynthia Cherry
978-1941070000

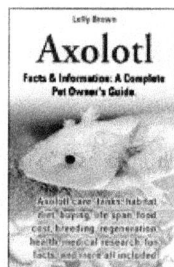

Axolotl
Lolly Brown
978-0989658430

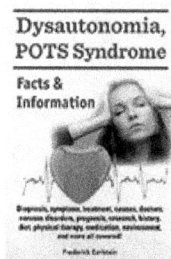

Dysautonomia, POTS
Syndrome
Frederick Earlstein
978-0989658485

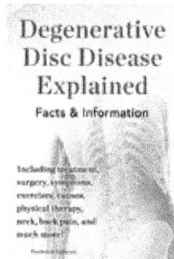

Degenerative Disc
Disease Explained
Frederick Earlstein
978-0989658485

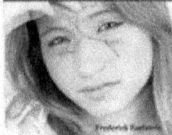

Sinusitis, Hay Fever,
Allergic Rhinitis Explained
Frederick Earlstein
978-1941070024

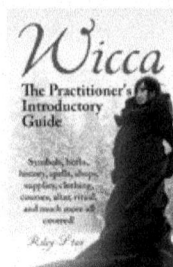

Wicca
Riley Star
978-1941070130

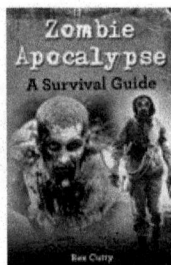

Zombie Apocalypse
Rex Cutty
978-1941070154

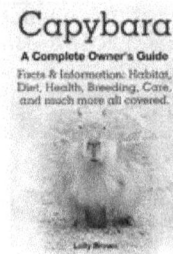

Capybara
Lolly Brown
978-1941070062

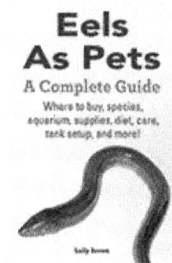

Eels As Pets
Lolly Brown
978-1941070167

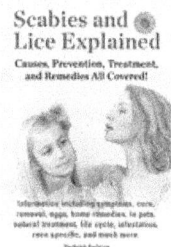

Scabies and Lice Explained
Frederick Earlstein
978-1941070017

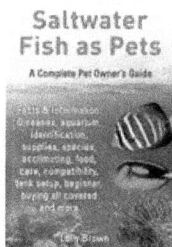

Saltwater Fish As Pets
Lolly Brown
978-0989658461

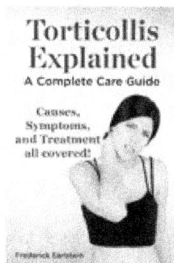

Torticollis Explained
Frederick Earlstein
978-1941070055

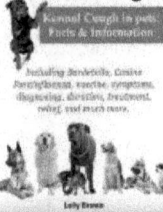

Kennel Cough
Lolly Brown
978-0989658409

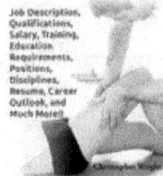

Physiotherapist, Physical
Therapist
Christopher Wright
978-0989658492

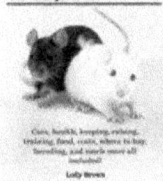

Rats, Mice, and Dormice
As Pets
Lolly Brown
978-1941070079

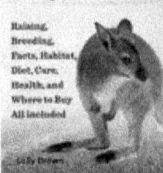

Wallaby and Wallaroo Care
Lolly Brown
978-1941070031

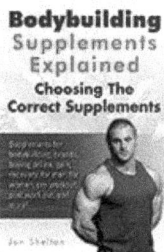

Bodybuilding Supplements
Explained
Jon Shelton
978-1941070239

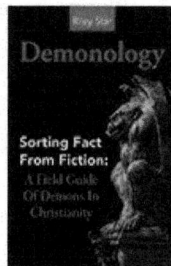

Demonology
Riley Star
978-19401070314

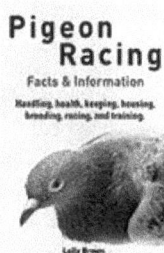

Pigeon Racing
Lolly Brown
978-1941070307

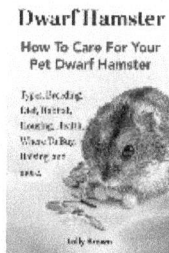

Dwarf Hamster
Lolly Brown
978-1941070390

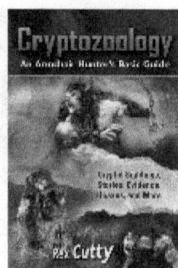

Cryptozoology
Rex Cutty
978-1941070406

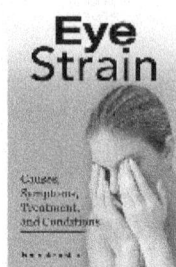

Eye Strain
Frederick Earlstein
978-1941070369

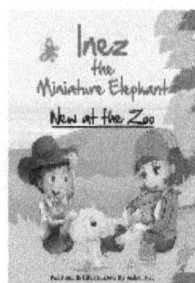

Inez The Miniature Elephant
Asher Ray
978-1941070353

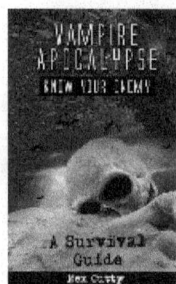

Vampire Apocalypse
Rex Cutty
978-1941070321

www.ingramcontent.com/pod-product-compliance
Lightning Source LLC
Chambersburg PA
CBHW062028200326
41519CB00017B/4974